How to Eat More Vegetables

A Concise Guide to
Help You Eat and Enjoy
the Most Important Food
for a Fulfilling Life

By Martin Meadows

Download Another Book for Free

I want to thank you for buying my book and offer you another book (just as valuable as this one): *Grit: How to Keep Going When You Want to Give Up*, completely free.

Visit the link below to receive it:

http://www.profoundselfimprovement.com/vegetables

In *Grit*, I'll tell you exactly how to stick to your goals, using proven methods from peak performers and science.

In addition to getting *Grit*, you'll also have an opportunity to get my new books for free, enter giveaways, and receive other valuable emails from me.

Again, here's the link to sign up:

http://www.profoundselfimprovement.com/vegetables

Table of Contents

Download Another Book for Free...................... 2

Table of Contents 3

Prologue 4

Chapter 1: Get Motivated to
Eat More Vegetables 8

Chapter 2: Which Vegetables
hould You Eat?.................................... 24

Chapter 3: How to Eat Vegetables
Every Day... 45

Chapter 4: Learn to Love Veggies 69

Chapter 5: Frequently Asked Questions
and Other Challenges 90

Epilogue 109

Download Another Book for Free.................. 111

Could You Help?................................... 112

About Martin Meadows 113

Prologue

I want you to become a superhero.

To claim your superpower abilities, you don't need to travel to a remote temple high in the mountains and train for decades. All you need to do is invest a few weeks into creating a new habit in your life that will give you more energy, optimize your performance, and ultimately help you live a more fulfilling life.

What is this habit? It's proper nutrition, and more specifically, eating vegetables *daily*.

Food has an unbelievable impact not only on our bodies, but also our psychology. Optimizing your diet can have an immense impact on your life.

Take dark green leafy vegetables like Brussels sprouts, kale or spinach. Did you know that they're a rich source of folate which helps regulate mood and whose shortage is linked with depression?[1]

Little folate in your diet = little happiness in your life.

It isn't just dark green leafy vegetables that regulate your mood: all vegetables can help.

In a study on over 80,000 people, individuals who ate more fruits and vegetables felt happier and had a higher life satisfaction than people who didn't eat enough portions (well-being peaks at approximately 7 portions per day).[2]

Again, little veggies = little fun.

Now consider beta-carotene, a red-orange pigment found in large amounts in carrots, pumpkins, sweet potatoes, spinach and collards. Eating beta-carotene rich foods will give your skin a nice, healthy glow that most people think you can only get with expensive skin creams.

According to a small study conducted by psychologists at University of Western Australia, beta-carotene not only enhances your facial color, but also makes you more attractive and look healthier.[3]

The more veggies you eat, the better you look. How cool is that?

There are plenty of other surprising benefits of vegetables, but I think that you get the point:

vegetables are like Gummiberry Juice, the secret concoction gummi bears in the animated television series consumed regularly to gain superpowers that enabled them to escape from all sorts of troubles.

Yet, because so many people think that vegetables are unappetizing, expensive, hard to prepare, or otherwise challenging to consume, they don't eat even a quarter of what they should be eating.

The Centers for Disease Control and Prevention estimates that only nine percent of Americans met the intake recommendations for vegetables.[4]

Nine percent! It's incredible that vegetable growers aren't out of business yet.

Seven of the top 10 leading causes of death in the United States are from chronic diseases— diseases can be largely prevented with a healthy diet rich in fruits and vegetables.[5]

As a self-certified veggie addict and personal development writer, I had to write this book. It pains me that so many people lack energy, struggle with depression, obesity, high blood pressure and other unpleasant conditions largely because they lack key nutrients vegetables provide in spades.

If this book helps at least a handful of people, I'll be happy knowing that I made at least a small positive impact on the world.

Let's proceed to the first chapter addressing one of the biggest questions: how do you get motivated to eat more vegetables?

Chapter 1: Get Motivated to Eat More Vegetables

You know that eating vegetables is good for you. Yet, you don't eat them as often as you should. Vegetables being good for you is not a good enough reason to convince you to change your ways.

In this chapter we'll go through the most effective techniques to get yourself motivated to eat more vegetables. These techniques are simple, but don't let their simplicity fool you. Done right, they *will* inspire you to change your diet.

Technique #1: Identify What's Important to You

The argument that vegetables are good for you is weak because it fails to produce an emotional impact. Yes, you'll be healthier when you eat vegetables, but so what? How do the benefits apply *specifically* to you?

Start by identifying your most important values. Don't spend a lot of time on this exercise as I don't want to lose your attention. Five items are more than sufficient. Let's say that your top five most important things are:

1. Your family.

2. Your career or business.

3. Financial security.

4. Helping kids as a sports coach.

5. Playing golf.

Now that you have your list, it's time to create what I call a *motivational link*—a bridge between a new habit and your current set of habits.

The goal is to sell yourself the new habit by identifying how it can have an impact *specifically* on what you hold dear. Considering that we are talking about vegetables, it might be a strange exercise, but please try it: I'm sure that something will strike a chord with you. Here's how you can link the aforementioned top five items with eating more vegetables (adapt them to fit your unique circumstances):

1. Your family. You want to take care of your family. They want you to be vibrant and happy so that

together you can enjoy life to the fullest. Eating more vegetables will dramatically improve your health, make you more energized, and ready to serve your family on all levels even better than ever before.

2. Your career or business. You need to operate at maximum efficiency. You need to be productive and creative to ensure that your career or business constantly grows. A supercar needs high-quality fuel. *You* are this vehicle.

3. Financial security. It takes discipline to save money for your dreams and to be prepared for emergencies. Vegetables are not only cheaper than processed food: they're also more economical due to their highly nutritious content. One pound of leafy greens satisfies your body's needs for vitamins and minerals more effectively than a pound of processed and prepared snacks. Healthy eating will also help you protect yourself against some unpleasant and costly disorders—and with less money spent on medications, you have more money you can save for the future.

4. Helping kids as a sports coach. The kids you coach to become confident, healthy and athletic adults need you to be their mentor. Leading by example is the best way to inspire change in others. By eating more veggies you'll develop real-world nutritional knowledge to pass on to your proteges.

5. Playing golf. All professional athletes, no matter the discipline, pay close attention to their nutrition. If you want to finally lower your handicap this year, you need all the help you can get. Veggies can be one of your most powerful allies.

Can you see the difference that translating the benefits of eating vegetables to your own unique situation makes? What produces a more motivating emotional response: Vegetables are good for you, or eating more vegetables will help you serve your family on all levels even better than ever before?

A Side Note About Prevention

Please note that this technique is *not* about visualizing how you can prevent something bad from happening.

Despite prevention being better than cure, most people go to the doctor only when they feel unwell. A regular check-up could help identify early warning signs and prevent suffering. Unfortunately, preventive medicine is a hard sell because it aims to get people thinking about the future that might or might not happen.

The fact that 30,000 premature deaths per year in the United States are attributable to consumption of trans fatty acids,[6] which are found in donuts and many other unhealthy foods, won't make most people stop eating donuts.

That's why the most common arguments to encourage people to eat more vegetables don't work. Who cares about something that might or might not happen in the future? We already have enough things to worry about today.

While prevention obviously makes sense, using it as an argument to take action—unless a person already suffers from some negative consequences of their bad habits—fails to get people to act, so instead focus on techniques that aim to improve your life.

Technique #2: Motivation in Reverse

Many motivational approaches rely on pulling yourself toward a specific outcome, but what sometimes works better for some people is the opposite: motivating yourself by escaping from something.

As I've already emphasized it, prevention generally fails to motivate people who feel alright (thus far), so this technique primarily works if you already suffer from some negative consequences caused by a bad diet.

A smoker won't give up smoking merely because a pack of cigarettes comes with a health warning, but they may come to senses when their doctor asks them to sit down because they have bad news (hopefully with a good prognosis).

Likewise, a person staying away from vegetables is unlikely to suddenly start devouring pounds of broccoli just because somebody told them that an unhealthy diet may lead to a heart attack. Unfortunately, it's only when they experience chest pain that they finally remove their blinders and improve their diet.

To give yourself a burst of motivation, look at these early signs with a magnifying glass and visualize subsequent, even worse consequences that are bound to happen if you fail to act today. Think of it as engineering a significant emotional event in your mind and harnessing it to motivate you to take action before it turns into reality.

For example, if you devour hamburgers all day long and you're tired all the time, obese, and short of breath, there's no denying the fact that you're on track to develop a host of unpleasant conditions, courtesy of a bad diet.

Intensify this negative vision. Make it painful to watch. Now draw inspiration out of this gloomy vision. Realize that you can still make different choices. You can opt for a different path that will take you toward a more positive future.

Technique #3: Identify Your Allies

When we're stuck in our old ways, we often fail to identify that there are allies in our immediate environment who can help us get unstuck. Since we assume we're on our own, without access to any external help, motivation is hard to come by.

Identifying resources that can help you get on track can shake you out of inaction. The realization that there are people who can help you may inspire you to act.

Perhaps there's a colleague at work who lost a lot of weight last year and can give you some pointers and support. Maybe your spouse eats a lot of veggies, but you always rejected their offers of help. Possibly there's a group of people at your local gym who are working on changing their nutritional habits and would welcome you as a new member.

Think of people who can help you change your diet and reach out to them. With a feeling of support, you'll be more likely to make a move and finally incorporate more vegetables in your diet.

Technique #4: Create an Alter Ego

Okay, I'll admit it: this technique is unusual, but it's been one of the most paramount strategies that helped me improve my diet. I'm certain it can help you, too.

Let's start at the end, because that's the first step to execute this method. Imagine your perfect future. How would different areas of your life look so you could rate them a 10 out of 10?

What kind of a person would be able to enjoy such a life? What traits would he or she have? How would he or she act? What would be his or her habits?

Now let's backtrack their steps. How did they form these habits? What events or decisions made them act this way? How much time did they spend developing these traits and the lifestyle they now enjoy?

Answer these questions and create your alter ego: a new identity that you can adopt today to get yourself on the path toward your perfect future. Like in the first technique, make sure that it's clear why eating veggies is a key element of this perfect vision (hint: if your ideal alter ego is healthy, what is their diet like?)

From now on, ask yourself repeatedly: would the perfect Joe or Jane engage in this habit? Would they take this decision? Would they fail to take action?

Anytime you struggle with your new habit, remind yourself of this perfect vision and remember that every deviation from the ideal traits and habits puts distance between your present and the ideal future.

Technique #5: A Carrot and a (Celery) Stick

If you're strongly motivated to get a reward or to avoid punishment, consider coming up with a carrot (sorry, I couldn't resist) and a (celery) stick (I apologize for two bad jokes in a row; it won't happen again).

Eating more vegetables produces many rewards you'll soon experience, but if you aren't convinced about them, come up with an additional reward. For example, two weeks of eating vegetables every day gets you a massage or taking your family to the movies.

Your reward needs to be motivating, but can't produce effects that would jeopardize your new habit. For example, don't reward yourself with a big cake or a week without veggies after successfully eating them for the past two weeks. In other words, don't reward your virtues with vices: come up with pleasant activities that are exciting and good for you.

If rewards don't motivate you as much as potential punishments, set a penalty for failing to honor your promise. For example, you'll need to send $100 to an organization you don't support or spend an entire day taking care of all the household chores (your significant other or roommate will be happy to keep you accountable with this one).

Punishments as a safeguard to honor your commitment can work like magic but be careful not to put yourself under too much pressure. The penalty has to be uncomfortable and painful, but not so traumatizing that you'll never again even consider eating a single stalk of broccoli.

Commit to This Habit Today

If there's one decision that can help you eat more vegetables, it's committing to eating a specific amount of vegetables a day. Not every other day: *every day*.

Depending on your gender, age, and level of physical activity shoot for a half a pound (250 grams) to about a pound (a half a kilogram) of vegetables a day, which is roughly in line with the official recommended daily vegetable intake in many countries around the world.

Don't concern yourself with the number of servings or cups. It's a super confusing metric that makes everything needlessly complicated (who puts their veggies in a cup?).

Weigh your food with a kitchen scale until you learn to eyeball things. You can also look up the average weight of vegetables. Type: "what 1 pound of [insert vegetable] looks like" in Google and you'll quickly learn how to estimate your veggie intake.

Yes, consuming between a half a pound and a full pound of vegetables means that most of your diet will revolve around veggie. And that's how it should be if you want to live a healthy life and radiate with energy.

Strive to hit your target with a variety of vegetables. Make a salad with radishes, cucumbers, bell peppers, beans, and carrots. Cook a vegetable soup with cauliflower, broccoli, cabbage, and other green leafy veggies. Grill an eggplant or zucchini. Make a frittata.

After a big portion of vegetables, you'll feel full and less likely to indulge in unhealthy foods (this in itself is a super simple weight loss strategy). Within a few weeks, your palate will get used to vegetables. Soon, you'll develop cravings for veggies instead of the processed foods.

Keep in mind that half measures don't work here. Commit and prioritize vegetables in your menu. Track your habit: mark off days by putting an X on them until eating veggies becomes a natural part of your life.

Now that we've got motivation covered, let's talk about selecting the right veggies to add to your daily menu.

GET MOTIVATED TO EAT MORE VEGETABLES: QUICK RECAP

1. Identify what's important to you and think how eating more vegetables can help you enjoy these things even more. The goal is to create an emotionally-charged link that applies specifically to your life.

2. For those who have spotted some negative consequences of an unhealthy diet in their lives, focus on those issues, magnify them, and visualize your life with these problems. The more painful the vision, the stronger motivating impact it will have to change it.

3. Identify resources you have in your life that may help you start eating more vegetables. A lack of support can make a person reluctant to make a change. That's why identifying who can help you will inspire you to take action.

4. Create an alter ego: a perfect vision of yourself. Imagine how this person acts, what habits and traits she or he has, and what decisions he or she made to get where they currently are. Now realize

that you can become this person if you model your life after them.

5. Use a carrot and a stick, or in other words, receive a reward for eating more veggies or a punishment in case you fail to change your nutritional habits. A reward should be exciting and good for you; it can't jeopardize your resolution to eat healthier. A punishment should be severe enough that you're afraid of it, but it shouldn't cause trauma that will make you give up your goals.

6. Commit to a habit of eating a specific amount of vegetables every day. Your intake should be between a half a pound to a full pound so that your diet revolves mostly around vegetables. This way, you'll always feel full and quickly train your palate to enjoy and crave more vegetables. Half measures don't work: commit.

Chapter 2: Which Vegetables Should You Eat?

If you can get twice or thrice as many benefits with less effort, would you take this opportunity?

Of course you would.

And that's what you get if you focus on nutritionally-dense vegetables. In this chapter we'll go through 33 vegetables: 13 that don't have a rich nutritional profile and 20 that are most nutrient-dense.

Let's start by reviewing vegetables that offer a low return. They aren't necessarily unhealthy. Our goal is to get the most nutrients possible for the least amount of calories, so any vegetable that doesn't provide that is a low-return vegetable.

It doesn't mean that you should stop eating vegetables from the following list. You can get more benefits by eating different veggies, but variety is still important and if you enjoy any of the low-return vegetables, don't stop eating it.

Some vegetables featured in this chapter are botanical fruits, but they're considered culinary vegetables and so I treat them as such.

13 Low-Return Vegetables

The vegetables are listed in alphabetical order, and the list features only the most common ones.

1. Celery

Except for vitamin K and some vitamin B9 (folate), celery doesn't contain other nutrients in substantial quantities. Throw it in your soup or eat some celery stalks, but don't make it a staple of your diet.

2. Cucumbers

With peel, cucumber contains some vitamin K and trace amounts of other vitamins and some minerals. While it isn't packed with nutrients, it's low in calories so don't be afraid to eat it as much as you want—it's perfect in salads.

3. Eggplant

With the exception of manganese, eggplant isn't a rich source of key nutrients. For variety, by all means eat it if you like. If you're seeking a lot of nutrients packed in a single veggie, eggplant isn't it.

4. Green beans

Green beans do contain some nutrients like vitamin C, K, B6 and manganese. However, these nutrients are available in higher amounts in other vegetables. There's no harm in eating green beans, but if you want to maximize the positive effects of eating vegetables, there are better alternatives.

5. Iceberg lettuce

Iceberg lettuce contains fewer nutrients than darker or more colorful lettuce varieties like red leaf lettuce or kale. It works in salads, but don't make it the base of your salad as there are far better, more nutritious options.

6. Olives

Just 3.5 ounces (100 grams) of olives provides more than the daily recommended intake of sodium, which most people already get far too much.

Olives are a good source of vitamin E, though, so throwing some olives in your salad isn't a bad idea as long as you watch your sodium intake.

7. Onions

Onions are great for flavor and aroma, but don't offer much in terms of nutrition. They contain some vitamin C and vitamin B6 but are otherwise a poor source of nutrients.

8. Radish

Just like cucumber, radish isn't bad in itself. It just doesn't offer many nutrients, with vitamin C being the only exception. Radishes add crunch to your salads and can serve as a quick healthy snack, but other than that, they won't have a big impact on your health.

9. Spaghetti squash

When cooked, spaghetti squash has an interesting texture resembling spaghetti. And just like spaghetti, spaghetti squash isn't a particularly nutritious choice. If you're looking for a healthy alternative to spaghetti, spaghetti squash is a good option. When compared to other vegetables, it isn't the most optimal choice.

10. Sweet corn

Sweet corn is technically not a vegetable—it's a grain—but it's usually considered a vegetable. It's a good source of vitamin B1 (thiamine) and an okay source of vitamin B3 (niacin), vitamin B9, and magnesium.

The problem with sweet corn is that it's high in carbohydrates. The ratio of nutrients to calories isn't favorable for weight loss. Eaten occasionally, it probably won't harm you. If you're struggling with your weight, you can skip it for better options.

11. Tomatoes

Tomatoes are similar to cucumbers: they're great for salads or eaten raw, but otherwise don't provide much nutrients except for vitamin C. They're low in calories and have a nice flavor, so don't avoid them in your diet—just don't consider them a rich source of vitamins and minerals.

12. Turnips

Except for vitamin C, boiled turnips don't provide any other nutrients in substantial amounts.

Don't mistake them with turnip greens (leaves of the vegetable) which we'll discuss later.

13. White potatoes

Oh, the much beloved and hated white potato. Some don't consider it a vegetable, while others can't imagine their life without it.

What's wrong with white potatoes?

The main objection is that they're high in carbohydrates and have a high glycemic index meaning that they spike your blood sugar levels quickly. Research suggests that consuming low-glycemic foods is an effective method of promoting weight loss and improving lipid profiles[7], so if you often eat foods that spike your blood sugar levels, you may struggle with your weight.

Secondly, potatoes can be prepared in a wide variety of ways, many of which make it easy to overeat them (French fries, baked potatoes, etc.). Since potatoes, except for vitamin C, B6, and to a smaller extent, potassium and phosphorus, aren't nutritious, you don't get much value considering they provide so many calories.

The most sensible approach, assuming they don't cause any adverse effects in you, is to eat them in moderation if you cook them yourself. Completely eliminating white potatoes from your diet isn't a bad idea. Their absence in your diet won't harm you, and if you're struggling with weight, it may even help.

Top 20 High-Return Vegetables

Let's switch our focus to vegetables that offer the highest nutritional return.

If a vegetable you like isn't on the list, it's most likely because its nutritional profile wasn't rich enough. Asparagus is a healthy vegetable, but except for very high levels of vitamin K, it doesn't provide other nutrients in higher amounts.

Eat asparagus if you like. It's not a bad vegetable. If you're looking for the best option, however, it's better to eat broccoli or kale, which in addition to vitamin K, supply other nutrients in substantial amounts, too.

The vegetables are listed in alphabetical order, and the list features only the most common ones.

1. Arugula

Add arugula to your salads. It has a rich nutty flavor and smell and is loaded with vitamin K, A, C, and B9. It's also a good source of manganese, calcium, magnesium, and potassium. Don't overdo it, though: too much arugula in your salad will make it too bitter.

2. Beans

Beans provide more calories than other vegetables, but they're a great source of protein and dietary fiber. Some of the most common varieties of beans include black beans, chickpeas, pinto beans, adzuki beans, navy beans, and red kidney beans.

Since most beans have a similar nutritional profile, I decided to include them in the list as a group instead of listing them all individually. Depending on the variety, they supply high levels of vitamin B9, B1, and several minerals like magnesium, manganese, phosphorus, iron, and zinc.

Beans contain more sodium than other vegetables, so control your intake. If eaten dry, increase their digestibility by:

- soaking them for at least 10 hours,

- boiling for 5 minutes and letting them soak for a few hours,

- sprouting them.

3. Bell peppers

Bell peppers are low in calories and are one of the richest vegetable sources of vitamin C. They're also a good source of vitamin B6 and vitamin A (particularly red bell peppers). They're ideal for salads. Try red, yellow, orange, and green sweet bell peppers for a different nutritional profile and taste.

4. Broccoli

Broccoli is a rich source of vitamin C and K. It also provides in smaller amounts vitamin B9, B6, B5, B2 (riboflavin) and manganese. Boiling broccoli (and other cruciferous vegetables like Brussels sprouts, cabbage and cauliflower) ruins its anti-cancer properties[8], so make sure that you use other preparation methods, ideally steaming.

5. Brussels sprouts

Brussels sprouts supply high levels of vitamin K and C. They're also a good source of vitamin B9, B6, and B1 as well as manganese, and in smaller amounts, iron and phosphorus. They're also richer in protein than many other vegetables.

6. Cabbage

Cabbage is another good source of vitamin C and K. It also provides vitamin B9 and B6. Red cabbage in particular is worth the attention because unlike green cabbage, it's also rich in vitamin A and provides more vitamin C.

7. Carrots

Carrots are a powerful source of vitamin A, mostly in the form of provitamin beta-carotene. Consuming beta-carotene improves your skin color and is a method of sunless tanning, which I mentioned in the prologue. Carrots also supply small amounts of vitamin K and B6.

8. Cauliflower

Cauliflower has a high content of vitamin C and moderate levels of vitamin K, B9, B6, and B5. It's a versatile vegetable that you can use as an alternative for many unhealthy foods. For example, you can make cauliflower pizza crust or cauliflower bread.

9. Collard greens

Collard greens are one of the most nutritious cruciferous vegetables. They provide substantial amounts of vitamin K, are an excellent source of vitamin A (including beta-carotene) and are a good source of manganese, vitamin C, calcium, and vitamin B6.

10. Green peas

Green peas are a good source of vegan protein and contain moderate amounts of dietary fiber. They're more caloric than other vegetables on this list but worth it for all the nutrients they provide in high amounts: vitamin C, K, B1, manganese, vitamin B9, phosphorus, vitamin B3, B6, zinc, iron, and vitamin B2. Whew, what a list!

11. Kale

Kale is a superstar vegetable, and for a good reason. It's one of the richest sources of vitamin K and C, and supplies high levels of vitamin A, all B vitamins except for B3, and some vitamin E. It's also a great source of manganese and contains some calcium, magnesium, phosphorus, iron, and potassium. Eat it in a salad, prepare kale chips, or put it in your green smoothie.

12. Leeks

Leeks offer high amounts of vitamin K and manganese, and lower, but still substantial levels of iron, vitamin B6, B9, C, and A. You can add leeks to a wide variety of dishes, with vegetable soup being one of the easiest options.

13. Lentils

Lentils have the second-highest ratio of protein per calorie of any legume, after soybeans (which I don't include on this list given the nutritional controversies around soy).

Lentils are highly caloric and contain a lot of carbohydrates. However, their nutritional profile is exceptional. They are an excellent source of all B vitamins, and are loaded with iron, phosphorus, and zinc. They also provide in smaller amounts potassium and magnesium.

Unlike beans, you don't need to soak lentils, but you still can as it will reduce cooking time by half.

14. Microgreens

Microgreens are underdeveloped green leaves of leafy vegetables like broccoli, beets, kale, or arugula. They're harvested within about two to three weeks of planting and have higher concentrations of nutrients when compared to mature vegetables.[9]

Microgreens are different from sprouts (which are germinated in water) and baby greens (which are harvested after they develop the first set of true leaves but aren't quite full grown yet).

If you want to make your salad even more nutritious, go with microgreens over mature salad greens.

15. Quinoa

Quinoa, a staple South American food, is often mistaken as a gluten-free grain. In reality, it's a vegetable related to beets and spinach.

Cooked quinoa is an excellent source of manganese, phosphorus, and magnesium. It also provides some zinc, iron, and vitamin B9. Quinoa is a very rare vegetable source of protein providing all 9 essential amino acids.

Quinoa is more caloric than other vegetables, so treat it more as rice than a vegetable if you're on a weight loss diet. Try all three main varieties of quinoa for a different taste and a different nutritional profile: white, red, and black.

16. Romaine lettuce

Romaine lettuce is another vegetable that should often appear in your salads. It's a rich source of vitamin A, K, C and B9, while being very low in calories.

17. Spinach

Spinach is known for its high content of iron, but because of high levels of iron absorption-inhibiting substances, much of the iron in spinach is unusable by the body.[10]

While spinach won't help you with iron deficiency, it's still a highly nutritious vegetable supplying vitamin K in extremely high amounts. It's also rich in vitamin A, C, B9, B2, B6, E and minerals like manganese, magnesium, potassium, and calcium.

Popeye might not have been strong because of iron found in spinach, but other nutrients definitely helped.

18. Sprouts

Sprouts are seeds of vegetables germinated in water for a week. The most common sprouts include alfalfa, broccoli, soy, mung bean, sunflower, radish, soybean, and mustard. Similar to microgreens, sprouts are packed with more nutrients than fully mature vegetables.

The easiest way to add more sprouts to your diet is to put them in your salad. If you eat sandwiches, sprinkle some sprouts over them, too.

19. Swiss chard

Swiss chard provides extremely high amounts of vitamin K. It's also a good source of vitamin A, C, E, magnesium, manganese, iron and potassium. You can use fresh young leaves in your salads, while mature leaves are usually cooked.

20. Turnip greens

Turnip greens provide vitamin K, A, C, B9, B6, E, manganese, and calcium. They're also a good source of dietary fiber. Don't mistake them with turnips which are low in nutrients except for vitamin C.

Variety Is Important

Having listed produce with the highest and lowest nutritional return, I need to emphasize that the best strategy is to eat a wide variety of vegetables.

It isn't enough to pick just one or two highly nutritional vegetables. Pick at least five vegetables from the high-return list and eat them frequently. Don't stay away from the lower-return vegetables, either (perhaps except for white potatoes and sweet corn). While they aren't as high in nutrients, they still introduce more variety in your diet.

I don't want to delve too deep into nutritional science, but in addition to micronutrients like vitamins and minerals, vegetables also contain numerous other substances that are being investigated for their effect on human health. Eating various vegetables means getting a variety of substances that can potentially improve your health, so enrich your diet with different veggies.

A Word of Caution About Pesticides

The list of low and high-return vegetables doesn't address the fact that some vegetables are more contaminated with pesticides than others.

Each year Environmental Working Group releases its list of dirty dozen and clean fifteen produce, with the former being most contaminated with pesticides and the latter being least likely to be contaminated. The research assumes that the produce is peeled or rinsed as peeling and rinsing reduce the amount of pesticides.

As of 2018, there are five vegetables on the dirty dozen list (the rest are fruits):[11]

#2: Spinach—a staggering 97% of conventional spinach samples contained pesticide residues.

#9: Tomatoes—nearly four pesticides were detected on the average conventionally grown tomato.

#10: Celery—more than 95% of samples contained pesticides.

#11: Potatoes—they had more pesticide residues by weight than any other crop.

#12: Sweet bell peppers—almost 90 percent contained pesticide residues, with pesticides tending to be more toxic to human health than the ones found in other crops on the list.

If you consume these vegetables regularly, buying them organic would be best to reduce you and your family's exposure to pesticide residues.

And here are the vegetables on the clean fifteen list that you can largely buy conventionally-grown:[12]

#2: Sweet corn—less than 2% of samples had pesticide residues.

#4: Cabbages—14% of samples with pesticide residue.

#5: Onions— less than 10% of samples contained pesticides.

#6: Frozen sweet peas—about 20% of samples had pesticides.

#8: Asparagus—10% of samples had pesticide residues.

#10: Eggplant—about 25% of samples contained pesticides.

#14: Cauliflower—about 50% of samples had pesticide residues.

#15: Broccoli—30% of samples contained pesticide residues.

Now that you know both low and high-return vegetables, let's proceed to the heart of this book: how to eat more vegetables every day.

WHICH VEGETABLES SHOULD YOU EAT? QUICK RECAP

1. Low-return vegetables are vegetables that don't have a rich nutritional profile. They are healthy for you but won't have the biggest impact on your diet. Low-return vegetables include: celery, cucumbers, eggplant, green beans, iceberg lettuce, olives, onions, radish, spaghetti squash, sweet corn (you can skip it altogether), tomatoes, turnips, and white potatoes (you can skip them, too).

2. High-return vegetables are vegetables that have a diverse nutritional profile. They should form the majority of your diet. High-return vegetables include: arugula, beans, bell peppers, broccoli, Brussels sprouts, cabbage, carrots, cauliflower, collard greens, green peas, kale, leeks, lentils, microgreens, quinoa, romaine lettuce, spinach, sprouts, Swiss chard, and turnip greens.

3. For the maximum benefits, your diet should be varied. Pick at least 5 vegetables from the high-return list, but don't be afraid to eat low-return vegetables,

too (except for the ones that may have more drawbacks than benefits like white potatoes).

4. Be aware that some vegetables contain high amounts of pesticide residues. If it's possible, buy them organically grown. These vegetables include: spinach, tomatoes, celery, potatoes, and sweet bell peppers.

5. Some vegetables are low in pesticide residues and can be largely bought conventionally-grown. They include: sweet corn, cabbages, onions, frozen sweet peas, asparagus, eggplant, cauliflower, and broccoli.

Chapter 3: How to Eat Vegetables Every Day

As convenient as it would be to eat vegetables once a week and enjoy all their health benefits, unfortunately our bodies don't work this way. While the body stores some nutrients (for example fat-soluble vitamins and minerals), it doesn't store many others, like water-soluble vitamin C and B (except B12). This means that a healthy menu needs to feature vegetables every day, not just every now and then.

But how do you do it *daily* given how difficult and time-consuming preparing vegetables can be? This is what we're going to talk about in this chapter. Here are 11 methods to eat vegetables every day.

1. Eat Vegetables With Every Meal

The simplest strategy to eat more vegetables is to include them in every meal.

Duh.

I know. Still, it's one of the easiest strategies that requires only some tiny tweaks in your diet. Make a list of your favorite dishes. Go through them one by one and think how you can add some veggies to them. For example, if you often eat scrambled eggs, you can eat them with:

- spinach,
- a chopped bell pepper,
- raw cherry tomatoes as a side snack,
- asparagus,
- chopped zucchini,
- kale.

Google the name of your favorite dish and add "vegetables" at the end for countless ideas to upgrade your breakfast.

Another simple way to add vegetables to every meal is to make sure that each meal comes with any of the following:

- a salad (even if it's just a few spinach leaves with some cucumbers and radishes),
- some raw vegetables,
- soup as an appetizer,

- a vegetable smoothie (more on that later),

- veggie sauce like tomato sauce (make sure it isn't loaded with sugar),

- veggie spread or dip (like pesto),

- a greens supplement (this is the worst option, but if all else fails, at least you'll get some nutrients).

2. If You Snack, Snack on Vegetables

Snacking isn't beneficial for your health and weight. It's too easy to snack mindlessly, increasing your calorie intake well beyond what your body needs and with foods your body doesn't need.

If, however, you can't imagine your day without snacking, at least try replacing your usual snacks with some vegetables. No, I don't mean replacing popcorn with steamed vegetables or potato chips with soup. I talk about alternatives similar in texture, flavor, and appearance.

For example, there's nothing magical in potato chips that makes you snack on them so frequently.

Come on Martin, potato chips taste awesome!

Of course, they're cheap, addictive, and everybody loves them. However, if I gave you a

47

tastier and healthier alternative, wouldn't you make the switch willingly?

It's like with your daily commute: if I shared with you a faster and more convenient route, wouldn't you switch it in a heartbeat? Okay, daily commute isn't nowhere near as pleasant as eating potato chips, but I think you get the point: we often engage in certain activities because we aren't aware of better options or if we do, we don't give ourselves a chance to get to know them better.

If you never gave alternatives a chance, you can't assume that no healthy snack exists that's just as good as potato chips. If you enjoy snacking on potato chips, you can replace them with a vegetable alternative such as carrot chips, zucchini chips, or butternut squash chips (we'll discuss more options later).

Is it going to taste different? Absolutely. If, however, it's at least *almost* as good as the original, you *can* make the switch permanent if you give yourself some time to get used to the new flavor. That's what happened when I replaced white rice with quinoa. Its texture was strange at first, but once I ate it a few times, I got used to it.

There's no need to give up your favorite snacks right away. Make things easier by starting small. Replace potato chips with vegetable chips every other day or eat potato chips alongside with vegetables (for example, eat two carrots for each bag of potato chips). Give yourself time to get used to the new flavor and gradually switch from the unhealthy snack to a healthier alternative. Eventually you'll switch to veggie snacks or at least eat them more often.

If you find it impossible to replace your favorite snacks with vegetables, consider designating veggie snack days. As the name implies, pick at least one day a week (and ideally two or more) on which you're allowed to snack only on vegetables.

Since it's a tiny change, it shouldn't produce as much mental resistance as the idea of replacing all your favorite snacks with veggies.

3. Make Vegetables Your Passion

Or more specifically, make them a component of your passion.

If you enjoy jogging and usually follow it with a fruit smoothie, why not mix in some leafy greens like kale or spinach? You probably won't notice a big difference in taste (or there might even be an improvement), and just like that, you've consumed some vegetables with no big changes to your diet.

If you enjoy hiking, your menu doesn't have to consist exclusively of protein bars with artificial sweeteners. For some variety on your treks, you can take some carrots, celery sticks, homemade veggie chips, dehydrated vegetables, healthy protein bars made exclusively of vegetables, fruits, and nuts, or some green vegetable powder supplement to add to your drinks.

If you love watching movies and there's always popcorn by your side, slice some carrots, celery sticks, bell peppers, and cucumbers and serve them with a hummus dip.

If you enjoy cafés, coffees and cakes, consider going to a healthy vegan café where cakes are made from vegetables, fruits, and nuts. Yes, it's not a perfect source of vegetables, but a carrot cake is still better than your typical high-calorie sugary dessert devoid of any nutrients.

4. Double the Veggies

In most recipes that require vegetables, doubling the amount is an easy way to eat more vegetables without affecting the flavor. For example, omelets, casseroles, frittatas, quiches, and other similar dishes will taste equally good—if not better—with more vegetables.

The same applies to soups, which are richer and more filling if they aren't watery. Cream soups are excellent. You can blend several vegetables and as long as there's one that dominates, you probably won't even taste the addition of others.

Salads are the same—you would have to try very hard to ruin a salad by doubling the veggies. As long as you stick to vegetables from the same group as the ones featured in the recipe (for example, if the recipe calls for lettuce, you can safely add spinach, too), your salad will still be delicious.

5. Avoid Fancy Recipes

One of the most common reasons why people fail to eat enough vegetables is because they don't have time for or don't like cooking.

Let me share with you one thing about me: I'm hopeless when it comes to fancy recipes. Even if I read a new recipe over and over again, I'm still unsure how to follow it and doubt that the final result will be edible. Yet, I still eat a pound of vegetables a day and no, I don't eat out every day.

My super secret is that I stick to simple recipes. Preparation never takes me more than maybe 20-30 minutes. I don't like fancy recipes because in addition to a lot of prep time and often confusing directions, they often call for exotic things you don't even know where to buy. The effort required for these recipes isn't worth the result. If I want to eat something fancy, I eat out. If I want to provide my body with fuel, I cook a simple recipe (which still tastes good).

For example, I usually prepare the same salad, but with varying proportions of vegetables, herbs and spices. When I eat steamed vegetables, I have a few favorite vegetables and a couple of favorite sauces.

Since I follow a similar process each time, it's impossible to end up with an inedible result.

If you enjoy cooking, by all means try fancy recipes—chefs make the world a better place! Those of us who don't possess such skills or don't have time are better off sticking to simple recipes.

6. Cook Once, Eat for Days

Another strategy for busy people is cooking dishes that you can eat for several days.

Soups are one such example. It doesn't take much time to chop additional vegetables and have a meal for a few days. Soups often taste better the next day because the ingredients have a chance to mix properly and absorb the broth.

Stews and chilis are similar to soups in that they also taste better the next day. Frittatas, quiches, omelets, casseroles, ratatouille and similar vegetable-rich dishes also work well as a make-ahead dinner idea.

While fresh salad is best, you can keep it in your fridge for two or three days. To keep it from getting soggy, add dressing when you're ready to eat it.

You can also prepare a week of green smoothies, put them in a jar or a glass bottle, and freeze them. Each day, instead of having to prepare everything again, you can grab a smoothie from a freezer.

Google "cook once, eat all week" for countless dinner ideas that you cook once and eat for days.

7. Make Green Smoothies

Smoothies are usually prepared from pureed raw fruit with water, crushed ice, dairy products, nuts, and perhaps some sweeteners like honey, sugar, or stevia. To add more vegetables to your diet, you can blend some of them into your smoothie.

To avoid bitterness, up to 40-50% of your smoothie may come from vegetables. The rest should come from fruits and other ingredients. Switching from a fruit smoothie to a vegetable smoothie accomplishes three healthy things at once: it increases your vegetable intake, makes your smoothie more satiating due to additional fiber, and reduces your intake of fructose, a simple sugar found in fruits.

Raw leafy vegetables are best for smoothies. They include: beet greens, broccoli, kale, spinach, collard greens, Swiss chard, or parsley.

Selecting the proper vegetables and getting the proportions right can be tricky. If your first several smoothies are too bitter or otherwise unappetizing, you might be tempted to give up. That's why it's best to prepare your first green smoothies according to a proven recipe. Once you know how to prepare smoothies you enjoy, mix them up to better suit your taste buds.

8. Eat Frozen Vegetables

Fresh produce at your local supermarket may not be as fresh as you think. It's rarely (if ever) transported immediately after picking to the local supermarket. Much of the produce is imported from thousands of miles away. The longer it takes to get the vegetables to the store and then your home, the fewer nutrients will survive. In contrast, frozen vegetables are generally flash-frozen immediately after harvest. This process may affect some nutrients, but according to research, both fresh and frozen vegetables are healthy.

A two-year study comparing the status of selected nutrients (vitamin C, beta carotene, and vitamin B9) in broccoli, cauliflower, corn, green beans, green peas, spinach, blueberries, and strawberries has shown that there were no significant nutritional differences between fresh, frozen, and fresh-stored (five days of refrigeration) vegetables.[13]

Another study comparing the levels of vitamin C, B2, E, and beta-carotene in corn, carrots, broccoli, spinach, peas, green beans, strawberries, and blueberries has found that the vitamin content of the frozen produce was comparable to, and occasionally higher, than that of their fresh counterparts. The only exception was beta-carotene which decreased in peas, carrots, and spinach.[14]

Frozen vegetables provide a few big benefits:

- you don't have to worry about spoilage,
- you don't have to waste time cutting vegetables,
- you get different vegetables in smaller amounts.

When buying frozen vegetables, make sure they were flash-frozen immediately after harvesting. Except for pre-cutting, they can't be processed in any way before packaging as this process may alter their nutritional value.

Mixed frozen vegetables are one of the best options for a quick, healthy meal. You already have vegetables in the right proportions, and they're already cut, so all you need to do is steam them, add some herbs, spices and sauce, and you're good to go.

There are also ready-made frozen soup mixes which you cook right away or blend first and then cook.

9. Eat Canned Vegetables

Research conducted at Michigan State University compared nutrition and cost of select canned, frozen, and fresh fruits and vegetables. Their analysis has shown that nutrient scores were similar for all packaging options, with canned vegetables having a lower cost per edible cup compared to fresh and frozen vegetables. According to the researchers, canned vegetables can be a cost-effective and nutritious option of meeting daily recommendations.[15]

Research shows that canned tomatoes have more bio-accessible lycopene and antioxidants which makes them more nutritious than raw vegetables.[16]

Canned beans are more convenient and digestible when compared to dry beans. You need to soak the latter for at least a few hours to reduce their content of anti-nutrients, while the canned ones are good to eat right away.

One of the main concerns regarding canned vegetables is that many cans are manufactured with Bisphenol A (BPA), a synthetic compound which, according to the European Chemicals Agency, has endocrine disrupting properties (your endocrine system controls the hormones in your body).[17]

For this reason, it's best to choose brands that don't use BPA in their cans (canned vegetables sold in health food stores are usually from BPA-free manufacturers) or consume jarred vegetables.

Another issue is that some canned vegetables can be high in salt. If you have high blood pressure, this may be problematic. According to one study on canned corn, peas, and green beans, draining and rinsing of canned vegetables reduces sodium content by 9% to 23%.[18]

Does it mean that you should stay away from canned vegetables? Unless you need to reduce your sodium intake, eating canned vegetables can still be a viable option to increase your veggie intake. Make sure that you buy BPA-free cans and that the manufacturer didn't add sugar or other preservatives other than salt.

10. Subscribe to a Healthy Meal Delivery Service

Consider subscribing to a healthy meal delivery service: a service that delivers a meal kit (all the ingredients and a recipe) or ready-made meals. When you get vegetable-rich meals delivered to your door every day, you can no longer make an excuse that you don't have time to improve your diet.

Yes, at first sight it appears costly, but when you consider how much time you need to spend on grocery shopping, prepping and cooking, it might be cheaper to have your meals delivered.

If you aren't convinced, divide the weekly cost of the service by the number of hours you spend each week on these activities. For example, if it takes you on average 5 hours a week and the service costs $100, you can free up one hour of your time for $20. If you value one hour of your time more than $20, it can be a great solution to simplify your life and improve your diet.

11. Try This List of Vegetable-Rich Alternatives to Common Nutritionally-Poor Foods

The following list provides alternatives to some of the most common nutritionally-poor foods. By replacing at least some of these foods with their healthier counterparts you can increase your vegetable consumption.

1. Bread

- Eat Ezekiel bread which is made of sprouted grains and legumes.

- Eat corn tortillas (remember that corn isn't a particularly great option, but still better than white bread).

- In sandwiches, replace bread with slices of baked sweet potato or grilled eggplant.

- Use romaine lettuce for your sandwich wraps.

- Use raw tomatoes, bell peppers or cucumbers as the bun.

- Make butternut squash flatbread.

- Make cauliflower bread.

- Make farinata, a type of Italian flatbread made of chickpea flour.

- Whenever you eat bread, stuff it with as many vegetables as you can.

2. Pasta

- Cook spaghetti squash. While it isn't a particularly nutritious vegetable, it's still better than pasta.

- Try zoodles, thin slices of zucchini mimicking the look of pasta. Use a spiralizer to create spaghetti-like strands.

- Try shirataki noodles, which are made from the root of konjac, an Asian plant that has almost no calories, but is very high in fiber.

- Cook cabbage noodles.

- Try black bean pasta.

- Try green pea pasta.

- Try lentil pasta.

- Try chickpea pasta.

- Try rice alternatives.

- Whenever you eat pasta, add some vegetables to it (in addition to sauce).

3. Rice

- Quinoa. As we've already discussed, while quinoa is often mistaken as grain, it's actually a vegetable—and a highly nutritious one, at that. Try all three main varieties (white, red, black).

- Make cauliflower rice.

- Make broccoli rice.

- Make sweet potato rice.

- Try pasta alternatives.

- Rice and beans are a nice combination for a post-workout meal.

4. Pizza

- Try cauliflower pizza.

- Try zucchini pizza.

- Try quinoa pizza.

- Cook a frittata, an egg-based Italian dish slightly resembling pizza.

- If you like pizza mostly because of melted cheese and not the crust, you can recreate the taste with some vegetables and cheese sprinkled on them.

- Whenever you eat regular pizza, go with as many vegetables as possible.

5. Potato chips

- Try kale chips.

- Try carrot chips.

- Try zucchini chips.

- Try eggplant chips.

- Try butternut squash chips.

- Try lentil chips.

- Try quinoa chips.

- Try any other vegetable-based healthy chips you can find in a health food store (read the labels carefully).

- Roasted radishes can work as a crispy snack, too.

- Replace white potato chips with sweet potato chips for added nutrition.

- If you can't give up potato chips, choose the most natural option available, with no preservatives, flavor enhancers, and other unhealthy substances.

6. French fries

- Try baked green bean sticks.

- Try oven-roasted celery fries.

- Make carrot fries.

- Try grilled asparagus fries.

- Try baked zucchini fries.

- Try turnip fries.

- Make chickpea fries.

- Try eggplant fries.

- Eat French fries made of sweet potatoes.

- If you can't give up French fries, make them yourself.

7. Popcorn

- Try roasted chickpeas.

- Make cauliflower popcorn.

- Cut some raw vegetables like carrots, celery stalks, bell peppers, or cucumber and dip them in hummus (which is made of chickpeas).

- Eat baby carrots—raw or baked, sprinkled with some herbs and spices or cheese.

- Eat cherry tomatoes.

- Try French fries or potato chips alternatives.

Now you have plenty of ideas on which vegetables to eat, how to eat them every day, and even how to replace your favorite processed foods with vegetables. The only question that remains is: how to learn to love vegetables? That's what we're going to discuss in the next chapter.

HOW TO EAT VEGETABLES EVERY DAY: QUICK RECAP

1. Upgrade all your favorite meals to include some veggies. Alternatively, make sure that each meal consists of at least one of the following: a salad, raw vegetables, soup, a vegetable smoothie, veggie sauce, spread, or dip, or as a last resort, a greens supplement.

2. If you have a habit of snacking, snack on vegetables—or at least add some vegetables to your usual snacks. Don't be afraid to experiment. Try various alternatives. Chances are that there are healthier snacks that you'll find just as tasty (if not more) than your current favorite snacks.

3. Make vegetables a part of your passion—include them as a post-workout meal, take them with you when hiking, enjoy vegetable-rich desserts in a café.

4. Double the amount of veggies called for in a vegetable-rich recipe like omelets, casseroles, frittatas, or quiches.

5. Avoid fancy recipes that require too much time spent shopping and prepping. Stick to simple dishes you can easily modify with different proportions of vegetables, herbs, spices, or sauces.

6. Cook dishes that you can eat for days. It only takes a bit more time to cook double or triple the amount and have a meal for a few days.

7. Make green smoothies, which usually consist of up to 40-50% of vegetables (primarily green leafy ones), the rest being fruits, nuts, and other usual smoothie ingredients.

8. Frozen vegetables are just as nutritious as fresh vegetables, so don't be afraid to stock up on them. It will save you a lot of time and trouble.

9. Canned vegetables are a cost-effective option to eat more veggies. If you have high blood pressure or need to avoid sodium for other reasons, be vigilant because canned vegetables are higher in sodium. Avoid BPA-lined cans or consume jarred vegetables instead.

10. Healthy meal delivery services offer a convenient way to eat more veggies with no grocery

shopping, little prep, and often, for an attractive price considering how much time they can save you.

11. Replacing at least some of your favorite processed foods with their healthier counterparts is a simple strategy to eat more veggies daily.

Chapter 4: Learn to Love Veggies

I used to dislike cruciferous vegetables like broccoli and cauliflower. I found their smell unpleasant and their taste off-putting. Other vegetables weren't much different. If I ate vegetables, it was white potatoes (constituting most of my vegetable consumption), carrots, radishes, cucumbers, lettuce, and bell peppers.

Today, I regularly eat a variety of vegetables, including such favorites nobody likes including Brussels sprouts, cauliflower, and kale. In fact, I can't think of any vegetables I would find too repulsive to eat.

I'm not saying it to brag (Who would brag about liking vegetables? This is so boring!). I'm saying it because if I learned how to do it—through trial and error—you can do it, too. Fortunately, thanks to the tips we'll cover in this chapter, you can largely skip the trial and error part.

Unlike fruits, which have a sweet taste, vegetables often have a bitter flavor or otherwise taste different than sweet, salty, or savory processed foods. This presents a challenge for people who eat vegetables rarely and whose palate revolts when they try to change their menu.

Changing your perception of vegetables comes down to two steps:

1. Eat more vegetables.

2. Learn how to cook and season them.

The first step helps you get comfortable with the different taste, while the second step helps you improve the flavor so they're more to your liking.

I wish I could share secrets that would make you instantly fall in love with vegetables, but there are none. Retraining your palate is about consistently exposing yourself to new flavors until you learn to enjoy them.

In a study on 360 fourth and fifth-grade students (unfortunately I couldn't find any studies on adults), repeatedly tasting disliked vegetables increased the children's liking of them. The approach of weekly taste exposures to carrots, peas, tomatoes, and bell peppers was effective in approximately half of the participants. The number of children who reported liking or liking a lot a previously disliked vegetable was greater after eight or nine taste exposures.[19]

If you're reading this book, you probably aren't a fourth or fifth-grade student. As an adult, you have more self-discipline than a typical kid, so this approach should be more effective.

Eating vegetables regularly expands your nutritional comfort zone so to speak. Bite by bite, meal by meal, as vegetables appear more frequently in your menu, they cease to become an unpleasant novelty.

Think of it as starting a new workout routine. At first, every exercise is uncomfortable. The next day your muscles are sore, and you hate yourself. But if you continue exercising, in a few weeks your incredible body adapts and you're no longer suffering—and instead, start enjoying the exercise.

Eventually, vegetables you initially *made yourself* eat find their place in your diet. You no longer eat them because you forced yourself to—you've adapted to the new taste and now you eat them because you *learned to like them*—assuming that they're cooked and seasoned to your liking.

Speaking of which, let's begin with the first key to improving the taste of veggies which is that...

It's All About Herbs and Spices

Let me make it clear: I almost never eat unseasoned vegetables (except for raw veggies) and don't believe anyone should eat them without a healthy sprinkle of herbs and spices. There are two main reasons:

1. Herbs and spices dramatically improve the taste

Every vegetable tastes markedly better with some herbs and spices.

In some cases, seasonings make or break a recipe. For example, I can't imagine eating an unseasoned soup. It's black pepper, salt, bay leaves, onions, garlic, basil, thyme and other seasonings that make soup delicious. Likewise, bland steamed vegetables aren't particularly enticing to eat. Sprinkle them with some salt, black pepper, and Herbes de Provence, and you have a nice, tasty meal.

This isn't just my personal belief. Research also suggests that using seasonings can help you eat more vegetables.

In a study on rural high school students, recipes with herbs and spices increased high school students' preference for several vegetables, with most seasoned vegetable recipes chosen over those with oil and salt alone.[20]

A study conducted on 148 adults suggests that herbs and spices can be a useful tool to improve the enjoyment of fat-reduced foods. As researchers nicely put it: "Adding spices is a way to reduce fat intake without sacrificing hedonic liking."[21]

2. Herbs and spices are healthy

In a comprehensive review on the health benefits of herbs and spices written by Australian researchers, the authors state that: "The real challenge lies not in proving whether foods, such as herbs and spices, have health benefits, but in defining what these benefits are and developing the methods to expose them by scientific means."[22]

By adding herbs and spices to your vegetables, you're getting more value out of your veggies. The amount of seasonings is usually smaller than a teaspoon a dish, but you're still getting some additional nutrients with little effort.

What Herbs and Spices Should You Use?

Seasoning is highly personal. I like most herbs and dislike Indian spices, while you might avoid basil and oregano but enjoy hot Mexican spices that would burn somebody else's tongue.

Let's cover some common versatile herbs and spices. Don't be offended if your favorite seasoning is not on the list. Use it as a starting point. Venture out and try other seasonings, too.

1. Salt

Before we talk about its use as a condiment, we need to discuss an important caveat. Salt is the main culprit behind overconsumption of sodium. Too much sodium is one of the most prominent dietary risks for disease,[23] with high blood pressure being one of the most harmful outcomes. If you need to avoid sodium for health reasons, do *not* use salt.

If you're otherwise healthy, however, prioritizing vegetables in your diet will reduce the amount of sodium-rich processed foods you eat, thus letting you enjoy some salt in your veggies.

What's more, many vegetables contain some potassium, which balances out the negative effects of salt and helps lower blood pressure. While potassium doesn't give you a free pass to eat salt in unlimited quantities, adding salt to foods that contain potassium is safer than eating salty foods devoid of this nutrient.

According to the World Health Organization, adults should consume no more than 5 g of salt per day, which is under a teaspoon.[24] Fortunately, this amount is more than sufficient to improve the flavor of your veggies.

Salt works well for almost every vegetable. Use it for steamed vegetables, to season your salad, to make your soup more flavorful and in virtually any other vegetable-based dish.

2. Pepper

Pepper is often paired with salt, and just like salt, it's versatile. Whenever you add salt, add some pepper, too, and you'll intensify the flavor even more.

For best aroma and flavor, buy whole peppercorns and grind them as needed rather than use pre-ground pepper, which lacks intensity.

3. Basil

Basil is one of the most appreciated herbs in the world for a reason. It works well both as a dried herb and fresh.

Fresh basil is the main component of pesto sauces (more on sauces later) and works like a charm with tomato in various forms including tomato sauce and tomato-based salads. Dried basil is perfect for salads, pastas, and soups.

A fun fact: you can make fresh basil tea. It smells horrible, but tastes decent.

4. Herbes de Provence

Herbes de Provence is a mixture of dried herbs that usually consists of savory, marjoram, rosemary, thyme, and oregano (lavender leaves are sometimes added too, but the original recipe doesn't call for it).

Instead of listing all the ingredients separately, I decided to include them as a single mixture because it's the most convenient and versatile mix you can use in a wide variety of recipes.

I use Herbes de Provence in almost every single dish. It works best for grilled and steamed veggies, roasted root vegetables, pastas, tomato sauces, and salads.

A fun fact: to slightly increase the nutritional value of bread, you can make a delicious dipping sauce with the herbs and olive oil.

5. Parsley

Parsley tastes best fresh, though its dried version is also available and can serve as a less flavorful substitute.

Its mild herbal flavor has numerous uses, with salads and soups being the most common dishes that benefit from its presence. You can also sprinkle some fresh parsley on hummus or when eating a vegetable-rich omelet or casserole.

6. Dill

As parsley, dill is best consumed fresh, though unlike parsley, its dried form isn't a bad alternative. In both forms, dill works well with potatoes, tomatoes, and cucumbers. You can use it for salads or soups, too.

7. Chives

Chives taste best when fresh, but dried chives are a good option, too. They work well with vegetable salads and egg-based vegetable-rich dishes.

8. Onions

Add sautéed onions to your veggies to enrich the flavor and make your dish more aromatic. Onions are also a staple component of soups. You can also use onion powder in your salad dressings.

9. Garlic

Available both fresh and dried, it's best to stick with fresh. Crush it, mince it, purée it, or roast it. You can use it for salad dressings, sauces, soups, stews, and many other dishes to achieve a richer flavor and aroma. It protects you against vampires, too.

10. Bay leaves

Bay leaves, both fresh and dried (with fresh being more flavorful than dried), work best for soups and stews. They imbue the dish with a subtle flavor and fragrance. They work well with tomatoes, beans, corn, and potatoes.

11. Cayenne pepper

If you like spicy food, cayenne pepper should be a staple in your kitchen. Cayenne pepper improves the flavor of stews, bean-based dishes, curries, and chilies.

12. Chili powder blend

Chili powder is a blend of spices composed of ground chili peppers and other spices, usually including cumin, garlic powder, onion, and sometimes salt. If you want to add piquancy to your vegetable dishes, this blend makes the job easy.

13. Paprika

Paprika is made from dried bell peppers. It adds a sweet and spicy flavor. Use it in soups, stews, casseroles and rice dishes.

There are dozens of additional common herbs and spices and thousands more less common, but the ones we've just gone through are a good start for a variety of applications and flavors.

Does it mean that now you need to buy all thirteen of them? Not really. Except for salt and black pepper, which you probably already have anyway, the decision to buy other seasonings depends on what you cook most frequently.

While I encourage you to experiment with single herbs and spices, consider purchasing a few different mixtures of dried herbs or spice blends. Chili powder blend will make your dishes spicy, while Herbes de Provence will permeate your veggies with an aromatic, herby flavor.

Go to the store, look at a few different mixtures and blends, check the ingredients (make sure that the mix doesn't have any artificial flavor enhancers), and experiment.

Just to show you what I personally use, here are the mixtures I use most frequently:

1. Garlic powder, parsley, salt, basil, onion powder, ginger, thyme.

2. Savory, onion powder, turmeric, tarragon, thyme, salt, basil, garlic powder, nutmeg, black pepper, allspice.

3. Herbes de Provence (we've already covered this one).

4. Salt, rosemary, thyme, paprika, pink pepper, savory, basil, tarragon.

5. Black pepper, chili, salt, coriander, white mustard, garlic powder, paprika.

Don't Forget the Sauce

Like herbs and spices, adding sauce to your dishes not only improves the flavor and taste, but also increases the amount of nutrients you get from your meal.

You can easily find ideas for hundreds of sauces online. Here, to get you started, we'll cover five simple versatile vegetable-based sauces.

1. Tomato sauce

The king of all sauces. It's easy to make it yourself, but if you aren't in the mood, buy it in a store. Make sure that your store-bought sauce doesn't contain any artificial enhancers.

Tomato sauce works well with pastas, beans, pizza, and Mexican-style recipes, but I use it for steamed vegetables, too.

2. Pesto

This basil-based sauce is usually made of basil leaves, crushed garlic, pine nuts, coarse salt, Parmesan cheese and pecorino sardo (cheese made from sheep's milk). The ingredients are then blended with olive oil.

You can make your own pesto, but it's more time-consuming than making tomato sauce. Pesto is perfect for pastas, but you can also add it to pizzas, salad dressings, or to garnish your vegetables instead of butter.

3. Spinach sauce

You can make spinach sauce with a lot of different ingredients. I usually make it with frozen chopped spinach, butter, and grated cheese (like Parmesan) or blue cheese (like Roquefort). Add garlic powder for additional flavor.

I mostly use spinach sauce to improve the taste of steamed vegetables, but its primary use is for pastas.

4. Salsa

Mexican salsa is a piquant tomato-based sauce usually including onions, chilies, and herbs. Use it for any vegetable dishes you'd like to spice up. It goes well with beans.

5. Garlic sauce (toum)

Toum is a Lebanese sauce made of garlic, olive or vegetable oil, and lemon juice. It's perfect for grilled vegetables. You can use it instead of mayonnaise.

Try Different Types of Cooking

Another simple way to alter the taste of vegetables is to try different types of cooking. For example, I find boiled vegetables less flavorful than steamed vegetables. For you, the taste of steamed vegetables might leave something to be desired and you might prefer grilled veggies. Different types of cooking and the resulting different textures can help you learn to like vegetables you would otherwise avoid.

Here are the main ways you can consume vegetables. Experiment with each of them.

1. Eat them raw

Eat them plain, like a rabbit. Dip them in sauce for improved flavor or put them in a salad.

2. Boil them

Unless you're making soup or stew, skip boiling and choose steaming.

3. Steam them

Less nutritional value is lost with steaming than with boiling, so it's a healthier way of cooking your veggies. Steaming is my default method of cooking vegetables.

4. Fry them

Without getting into an argument about what sautéing, stir-frying and pan-frying means, it's best to fry your vegetables using a low amount of fat so that you don't inadvertently double your calorie intake.

5. Roast them

Coat your vegetables with some oil so that they brown nicely. As with frying, don't go overboard with the fat. Works best with root vegetables like potatoes (choose sweet potatoes over white potatoes) or carrots. Zucchini, eggplant, and bell peppers are delicious roasted, too.

6. Grill them

Caramelized vegetables are more flavorful than steamed vegetables. Works best for vegetables like corn, eggplant, zucchini, asparagus, and bell peppers.

7. Purée them

Blend vegetables in your smoothie or make puréed vegetable soup. This makes veggies easier to digest.

8. Pickle them

Pickling is a form of fermentation that makes vegetables a good source of probiotics beneficial for the gut.[25] Sauerkraut (fermented cabbage), pickled cucumbers, and kimchi are some examples of fermented veggies. It's an acquired taste.

Periodically go back to vegetables you didn't find tasty and prepare them in a different way. As your palate changes, you may start enjoying foods that you've previously found bland.

Three Simple Steps to Tasty Salads

Eating a salad every day is one of the simplest ways to add more veggies to your diet. The key to tasty salads is the right dressing. I never use fancy dressings in my salads (store-bought thick salad dressing is usually unhealthy anyway). Instead, I default to the following three step process to make simple vinaigrette:

1. Add olive oil

For the best flavor, splurge a little and buy high-quality olive oil. If you want to go all nerdy, use the NYIOOC World Olive Oil Competition database at BestOliveOils.com to find the world's best extra virgin olive oils (don't worry, high-quality olive oil doesn't have to be prohibitively expensive).

2. Add acid

Vinaigrette is a mixture of oil and something acidic, usually three parts of oil to one part of acid. I usually use balsamic vinegar—as with olive oil, quality matters—but you can also use other types of vinegar (like apple cider vinegar) or lemon juice.

3. Add herbs and spices

Start with salt and pepper, and then add other herbs and spices to taste. I usually use a Mediterranean-style mixture of herbs including basil, thyme, oregano, rosemary, parsley, savory, marjoram as well as other mixtures with garlic and onion powder.

Now that we've covered various ways of learning how to love veggies, it's time for the final chapter that will answer some of the most commonly asked questions.

LEARN TO LOVE VEGGIES: QUICK RECAP

1. The two steps to learn to love veggies are: train your palate by eating more vegetables and learn how to cook and season them to your liking.

2. Herbs and spices are key to improving the flavor. Some of the most versatile seasonings include: salt, pepper, basil, Herbes de Provence, parsley, dill, chives, onions, garlic, bay leaves, cayenne pepper, chili powder blend, and paprika.

3. The second way to make vegetables taste better is adding sauce. Virtually all vegetable-based dishes will taste better with sauce. Some versatile sauces include: tomato sauce, pesto, spinach sauce, salsa, and garlic sauce (toum).

4. Another simple way to alter the taste of vegetables is to try different types of cooking. The main ways you can consume vegetables include: eating them raw, boiling, steaming, frying, roasting, grilling, puréeing, and pickling.

5. The key to tasty salads is the right dressing. By far the easiest one is vinaigrette. Use three parts of oil

(like olive oil) to one part of acid (like balsamic vinegar or lemon juice). Then add some herbs and spices.

Chapter 5: Frequently Asked Questions and Other Challenges

In the last chapter of this book we'll answer the eight most common questions and challenges my readers shared with me when asked what they find most difficult about eating vegetables.

Find it difficult to eat vegetables without added fat like butter, cheese, or a dressing?

Adding fat to vegetables makes them tastier yet increases the amount of calories your meal provides. Fortunately, if you switch from highly-processed foods to vegetables—even with some added fat— you'll still consume fewer calories.

For example, a half a pound of broccoli provides about 75 calories. The same amount of pasta provides about 288 calories. With a teaspoon of olive oil, your broccoli meal will provide 105 calories. Even with a tablespoon, it will still provide far fewer calories than pasta: 194.

As with most things in life, balance is key. Here are some pointers how to find it:

1. Gradually lower the amount of fat you add to your vegetables until you feel a noticeable difference in flavor. You'll be surprised how little fat you need to improve the taste. Halving the amount of olive oil, butter or grated cheese is unlikely to dramatically alter the taste, while it *does* dramatically lower the calories.

2. In salads, go with vinaigrette instead of a thick store-bought salad dressing, which is often extremely caloric and full of artificial flavor enhancers.

3. Add more herbs and spices to your dishes. Fat isn't the only way to make your veggies more flavorful.

4. When adding fat, think quality over quantity. Buy high-quality cheese—not the cheapest grated cheese—and you won't need to bury your veggies with it to enjoy a richer taste. The same applies to olive oil.

5. Add an avocado to your vegetables. It's high in fats, but richer in nutrients than olive oil or butter. Avocado is perfect for salads.

6. Experiment with low-calorie sauces like tomato sauce, which provide few calories, but change the flavor a lot.

Find it hard to prepare vegetables so they are easy to grab and go?

Here are 13 ideas for easy grab and go vegetables:

1. Munch on raw vegetables like carrots, bell peppers, cucumbers, or celery sticks. You can buy some of them, like carrots, peeled and pre-cut.

2. Make homemade veggie chips.

3 Make or buy dehydrated vegetables for a convenient quick snack.

4. Buy healthy protein bars made exclusively of vegetables, fruits, and nuts. Make sure they're free of sweeteners and other undesirable, unpronounceable ingredients.

5. Make a green smoothie.

6. Make a bread-free sandwich wrapped in romaine lettuce.

7. Bake green peas or buy them packaged. Add salt for taste.

8. Make a salad and pack it in a jar. Keep dressing in a separate container and add it later to prevent the salad from getting soggy.

9. Cherry tomatoes are a good portable snack, too.

10. Buy lentil or quinoa chips. Make sure they don't contain any artificial enhancers.

11. Roast vegetables ahead. They're good cold, too.

12. Pizza (not the best choice) and pizza alternatives (a much better choice) are okay to eat cold, too.

13. Make a cold soup like gazpacho.

Want your favorite comfort foods? Not in the mood to eat vegetables?

Unless you suffer from a mental disorder (wherein you *must* seek professional help), you're largely in control over how you feel.

If there's one thing that separates those who attain their goals from those who fail it's that the former take action even if they aren't in the mood. By taking action, those successful people *engineer* a mood conducive to positive changes. They refuse to delegate responsibility for their lives to something as fickle and finicky as their mood.

Eating vegetables is the same. I'm not always in the mood to eat healthy foods, either. However, I always make sure to eat them before I eat anything else. Often, this one action alone changes my mood. It's like exercising even when you don't feel like doing it—it usually lifts your spirits once you get started as it feels good to take care of yourself.

Even if eating vegetables doesn't improve my mood and, in the end, I still eat something unhealthy, at least I've already filled my stomach with some veggies and will eat less of the unhealthy foods.

Struggling with variety? Want to keep vegetables interesting?

Here are some ideas on how to avoid boredom when eating veggies:

1. The easiest way to keep vegetables interesting is to pair them with different herbs, spices, and sauces. For example, if you usually use salt, pepper, basil, thyme, and oregano to season your broccoli, try a chili powder blend to spice up your leafy greens. If you usually use tomato sauce, try other sauces, even if you don't think they'll work with your dish. Sometimes exotic combinations result in excellent recipes.

2. Try different types of cooking. For example, I usually make salads or eat steamed vegetables, but today I roasted a few different types of zucchini. The resulting flavor was different from what I usually eat, and now I have another simple recipe whenever I get bored of the meals I eat most frequently.

3. Regularly try new vegetables or a vegetable you haven't eaten for years.

4. Try all colors of the rainbow: if you usually eat red bell peppers, try orange, yellow, and green ones. If you usually buy green zucchini, try the yellow variety. If you're a fan of romaine lettuce, try the red one.

5. When making salads, experiment with proportions and use a different base vegetable. If lettuce is the base leafy green veggie in your salads, experiment with spinach, kale, cabbage, or other varieties of lettuce.

6. Garnish your veggies with cheese (try pairing them with different cheeses like parmesan, blue cheese, goat cheese, sheep cheese, mozzarella, etc.), nuts and seeds (they add a crunchy texture), or dried fruits.

7. Use dipping sauces: hummus, salsa, mayonnaise, mustard, garlic sauce (toum), tamarind sauce, pesto, Greek yogurt dip, tartar sauce, and any other sauce that strikes your fancy. Even if the veggies stay the same, the sauce will transform your dish.

Frustrated that fresh vegetables spoil so quickly and hate wasting food?

If you regularly throw away fresh vegetables, then stop buying them. Frozen vegetables are as nutritious (or sometimes more) than fresh vegetables. Canned or pickled vegetables are an option, too. If you have leftover fresh vegetables in your fridge, make a big soup.

If you don't want to give up on fresh vegetables, choose the ones that stay fresh far longer than others. Here are some that will last for at least two weeks when refrigerated:

- beets,
- cabbage,
- carrots,
- celery,
- green bell peppers (red, orange, or yellow will last for a week to two weeks at most),
- parsnips,
- pumpkins.

And here are some that last long that don't need to be refrigerated:

- eggplant,
- garlic,
- onions,
- sweet potatoes,
- white potatoes,

- winter squash (including butternut and spaghetti squash).

Can't afford to buy more vegetables?

Consider the following ideas:

1. Buy at a farmer's market. Many small farmers cannot afford to be certified organic yet grow their produce naturally with no pesticides. You'll save money, buy local and reduce your exposure to harmful chemicals.

2. Frozen or canned vegetables are often cheaper than fresh. You can also store them for longer, meaning you won't throw away food and waste your money.

3. Buy fresh vegetables when they're in season. They'll be more affordable and more flavorful.

4. Stock up on long-lasting vegetables when they're on sale.

5. One creative idea to gain access to cheaper vegetables is to…grow them yourself. If you have a backyard, you're only limited by the space you have. If you live in an apartment, there are some veggies you can grow indoors or on the balcony, including:

sprouts, microgreens, herbs, tomatoes, salad greens, carrots, radishes, celery, bell peppers, and green beans. Tower gardening is an option to grow your own food even in a small apartment.

6. Consider eating vegetables an investment in yourself. Eating healthily can prevent you from developing diseases that are ultimately much more expensive, not to mention their impact on your life satisfaction. Ask yourself how you can shift some of your expenses into buying healthier food or create a side income stream.

If you're concerned about the price of organic vegetables, remember that you don't have to buy all organic vegetables. Refer to the clean fifteen list for veggies that you can safely buy conventionally-grown.

Even if you can't afford organic vegetables, it doesn't mean that you shouldn't eat vegetables at all. Non-organic produce might contain more pesticide residues, but it doesn't cancel their health benefits or affect their nutritional content.

According to a systematic review on organic and conventional foods, "The published literature lacks strong evidence that organic foods are significantly more nutritious than conventional foods. Consumption of organic foods may reduce exposure to pesticide residues and antibiotic-resistant bacteria."[26]

Whether you buy organic or conventionally-grown vegetables, always wash them under running water. If you're concerned about pesticides, you can use a vegetable scrubbing brush and peel all vegetables (though some are fine to eat with a peel, including cucumbers, potatoes, and squashes).

How to work vegetables into breakfast?

Here are some ideas:

1. Scrambled eggs or omelets go with bell peppers. Onions and tomatoes are another option. Season with chives.

2. In sandwiches, you can replace bread with a variety of vegetables. Some easy time-efficient choices include sliced raw tomatoes, bell peppers, or cucumbers. You can also use romaine lettuce for your

sandwich wraps. If you don't want to give up bread, then add as many veggies to your sandwiches as you can: cucumbers, radishes, bell peppers, tomatoes, sprouts, carrots, spinach, lettuce. Sprinkle with fresh parsley.

3. For a light quick breakfast, dip raw veggies in hummus.

4. Add beans, peppers, olives, tomatoes, onions, and some leafy green vegetable like kale or spinach to your burritos.

5. If you eat pancakes, fill them with your favorite vegetables.

6. Make a green smoothie—as your main breakfast or to accompany your non-vegetable-based breakfast.

7. If you make hash browns or home fries, make them with more nutritious sweet potatoes instead of white potatoes.

8. You can add vegetables with a neutral or weak flavor to your oatmeal. Examples include minced zucchini, carrots, or puréed squash. Mince or purée

any vegetables you add to the oatmeal so that they mimic the size of oats.

9. Steam some veggies and eat them with fried eggs.

10. Skip breakfast altogether and eat a bigger meal later on. If you're concerned that skipping breakfast is unhealthy, read about intermittent fasting (a style of eating that cycles between periods of eating and non-eating).

In a 2014 scientific review of fasting, researchers concluded that "there is great potential for lifestyles that incorporate periodic fasting during adult life to promote optimal health and reduce the risk of many chronic diseases, particularly for those who are overweight and sedentary."[27]

Vegetables give you digestive problems?

There are many reasons why vegetables can give you digestive problems. Here are a few ideas to investigate:

1. If your body isn't used to lots of vegetables and dietary fiber, you might initially experience digestive problems. Letting your gut gradually

acclimate to a new diet over time can help prevent some discomfort.

2. If you always experience digestive problems after a particular vegetable (for example, broccoli), cut back on its consumption to see if it helps. No matter how healthy the vegetable is, if it doesn't work with your gut, it isn't worth it to eat it.

3. Eat more slowly. Vegetables are rich in dietary fiber and are harder to break down in your mouth and stomach than processed foods like pasta or white bread. Chewing more thoroughly, taking smaller bites, and eating more mindfully can help you eliminate issues caused by partially-digested foods.

4. Consider adding probiotics—helpful bacteria that aid in digestion—to your diet. The most common food source of probiotics are yogurt, kefir (fermented milk drink), and pickles (pickled in salty water and fermented—pickles made with vinegar don't contain live probiotics). You can also try sauerkraut, tempeh, kimchi, kombucha and miso.

5. Soak your beans when buying them dry to remove some of the oligosaccharides that cause

flatulence. Prior to eating canned beans, rinse them thoroughly.

6. Try to cook your vegetables in a different way. Perhaps roasted veggies give you problems, but steamed are fine. I myself don't feel well after eating fried vegetables, so I eat steamed or roasted vegetables instead.

7. Make green smoothies the primary source of your veggies. Blended vegetables are essentially pre-digested, which means they're unlikely to cause digestive problems.

If you experience frequent digestive problems regardless of your vegetable intake, please talk with your physician.

FREQUENTLY ASKED QUESTIONS AND OTHER CHALLENGES: QUICK RECAP

1. To find the right balance between adding fat to your veggies and making them too caloric, consider:

- gradually lowering the amount of fats until you notice a big difference in taste,

- in salads, choosing homemade vinaigrette over a store-bought dressing,

- adding more seasonings,

- adding less fat, but of higher quality,

- adding an avocado to your salads,

- experimenting with low-calorie sauces.

2. Some easy to grab and go veggie ideas include: raw veggies, homemade veggie chips, dehydrated veggies, vegetable-rich protein bars, smoothies, sandwiches wrapped in romaine lettuce, baked green peas, cherry tomatoes, lentil or quinoa chips, cold roasted vegetables, cold pizza and pizza alternatives, and cold soups stored in a jar.

3. If you aren't in the mood to eat vegetables, do it anyway. You're in control over how you feel—and

eating veggies can help you feel better even if you don't feel like doing it.

4. To keep vegetables interesting, consider:

- experimenting with different herbs, spices, and sauces,

- trying different types of cooking,

- experimenting with new vegetables regularly,

- trying different varieties of vegetables you already eat,

- experimenting with proportions in your salads,

- garnishing your veggies with cheese, nuts, seeds, or dried fruits,

- using dipping sauces.

5. If you regularly throw away fresh vegetables, then switch to frozen, pickled or canned veggies. When buying fresh veggies, focus on vegetables that last long in the fridge or that you eat frequently.

6. To optimize your expenses, consider buying at a farmer's market, buying frozen, canned, or pickled veggies, buying veggies when they're in season, stocking up on long-lasting vegetables when they're on sale, and growing veggies by yourself. Remember

that a healthy diet is an investment in yourself and diseases are more costly than vegetables.

If you can't afford to buy organic vegetables, realize that while conventionally-grown produce may contain more pesticide residues, it's still nutritious and definitely healthier for you than not eating veggies at all.

7. Make some small tweaks to your usual breakfast meals to make them vegetable-rich.

Eggs work well with bell peppers, onions, and tomatoes. Replace bread with raw vegetables as the bun or if you don't want to give up bread, add as many veggies to your sandwich as you can. Eat raw veggies dipped in hummus. Put vegetables in your burritos and pancakes. Have a green smoothie as your light breakfast. Make your potato-based breakfasts with more nutritious sweet potatoes. Add veggies with a neutral or weak flavor to your oatmeal. Serve steamed veggies with fried eggs. You can also consider skipping breakfast altogether and eating a bigger meal later on.

8. If vegetables give you digestive problems, a few potential solutions to try include:

- gradually increasing your vegetable intake so your gut can get used to higher amounts of dietary fiber,

- cutting back on the consumption of a vegetable that gives you problems,

- eating more slowly to better digest the veggies,

- adding probiotics like yogurt, kefir, pickles or sauerkraut to your diet,

- soaking your beans,

- cooking your veggies in a different way to see if the method of preparation affects your issues,

- making green smoothies the primary source of your veggies.

Epilogue

I sometimes think that I should price my books much, much higher than I do. No, it's not because I think that I'm the most awesome writer in the world. It's because I've found that the number of people who take action on the information they receive increases with the price they paid for it.

You respect information when you pay a lot for it more than information you receive for a low price or for free.

I'd hate for you to finish this book, feel self-congratulatory that you read it, and then never act on it. The title of this book is *How to Eat More Vegetables* for a simple reason: that's the goal I want to help you achieve. Try as you might, you can't achieve it by consuming *information*: you need to consume *the actual vegetables*.

If you could remember only two things from this book, please remember that:

1. Eating vegetables is a habit you develop through *commitment*. Today, commit to eating a

specific amount of vegetables and track your daily performance. If you merely resort to mental notes, you'll promptly forget about your resolutions and fail.

2. Learning to love veggies takes time, but *everybody* can train themselves to do it. Open your mind to new flavors, try different vegetables, use different herbs and spices, test different types of cooking, eat fresh, frozen, canned, and pickled vegetables, add various vegetables to your meals in all forms. Treat it as a fun experiment.

Your health is paramount to your enjoyment of life.

While you can't control everything that happens to your body, you are in control over your diet and can take actions that reduce the risk of preventable diseases. More energy, better appearance, and mental performance won't hurt either, will they?

Manifest your devotion to your loved ones and to *yourself* by eating vegetables every day. You only stand to gain.

Download Another Book for Free

I want to thank you for buying my book and offer you another book (just as valuable as this one): *Grit: How to Keep Going When You Want to Give Up*, completely free.

Visit the link below to receive it:

http://www.profoundselfimprovement.com/vegetables

In *Grit*, I'll tell you exactly how to stick to your goals, using proven methods from peak performers and science.

In addition to getting *Grit*, you'll also have an opportunity to get my new books for free, enter giveaways, and receive other valuable emails from me.

Again, here's the link to sign up:

http://www.profoundselfimprovement.com/vegetables

Could You Help?

I'd love to hear your opinion about my book. In the world of book publishing, there are few things more valuable than honest reviews from a wide variety of readers.

Your review will help other readers find out whether my book is for them. It will also help me reach more readers by increasing the visibility of my book.

About Martin Meadows

Martin Meadows is a bestselling personal development author, writing about self-discipline and its transformative power to help you become successful and live a more fulfilling life. With a straight-to-the point approach, he is passionate about sharing tips, habits and resources for self-improvement through a combination of science-backed research and personal experience.

Embracing self-control helped Martin overcome extreme shyness, build successful businesses, learn multiple languages, become a bestselling author, and more. As a lifelong learner, he enjoys exploring the limits of his comfort zone through often extreme experiments and adventures involving various sports and wild or exotic places.

Martin uses a pen name. It helps him focus on serving the readers through writing, without the distractions of seeking recognition. He doesn't believe in branding himself as an infallible expert (which he is not), opting instead to offer suggestions and solutions as a fellow personal growth experimenter, with all of the associated failures and successes.

You can read his books here:

http://www.amazon.com/author/martinmeadows

[1] Coppen, A., & Bolander-Gouaille, C. (2005). Treatment of depression: Time to consider folic acid and vitamin B12. *Journal of Psychopharmacology*, *19*(1), 59–65. doi: 10.1177/0269881105048899.

[2] Blanchflower, D. G., Oswald, A. J., Stewart-Brown, S. (2012). Is Psychological Well-being Linked to the Consumption of Fruit and Vegetables? *NBER Working Paper No. 18469*. doi: 10.3386/w18469.

[3] Foo, Y. Z., Rhodes, G., Simmons, L. W. (2017). The carotenoid beta-carotene enhances facial color, attractiveness and perceived health, but not actual health, in humans. *Behavioral Ecology*, 28(2), 570–578. doi: 10.1093/beheco/arw188.

[4] Lee-Kwan, S. H., Moore, L. V., Blanck, H. M., Harris, D. M., Galuska, D. (2017). Disparities in State-Specific Adult Fruit and Vegetable Consumption — United States, 2015. *Morbidity and Mortality Weekly Report*, 66(45), 1241–1247.

[5] CDC/National Center for Health Statistics (2017, March 17). Leading Causes of Death. Retrieved August 9, 2018 from https://www.cdc.gov/nchs/fastats/leading-causes-of-death.htm.

[6] Ascherio, A., Willett, W. C. (1997). Health effects of trans fatty acids. *The American Journal of Clinical Nutrition*, 66(4), 1006S–1010S. doi: 10.1093/ajcn/66.4.1006S.

[7] Thomas, D., Elliott, E. J., Baur, L. (2007). Low glycaemic index or low glycaemic load diets for overweight and obesity. *Cochrane Database of Systematic Reviews*. doi: 10.1002/14651858.CD005105.pub2

[8] Thornalley, P. (2007, May 15). Research Says Boiling Broccoli Ruins Its Anti Cancer Properties. Retrieved July 17, from https://warwick.ac.uk/newsandevents/pressreleases/research_says_boiling/.

[9] Xiao, Z., Lester, G. E., Luo, Y., & Wang, Q. (2012). Assessment of Vitamin and Carotenoid Concentrations of Emerging Food Products: Edible Microgreens. *Journal of Agricultural and Food Chemistry*, 60(31), 7644–7651. doi: 10.1021/jf300459b

[10] Savage, G. (1999). Oxalate content of foods and its effect on humans. *Asia Pacific Journal of Clinical Nutrition*, 8(1), 64–74. doi:10.1046/j.1440-6047.1999.00038.x

[11] Dirty Dozen. EWG's 2018 Shopper's Guide to Pesticides in Produce™. Retrieved July 14, 2018 from https://www.ewg.org/foodnews/dirty-dozen.php.

[12] Clean Fifteen. EWG's 2018 Shopper's Guide to Pesticides in Produce™. Retrieved July 14, 2018 from https://www.ewg.org/foodnews/clean-fifteen.php.

[13] Li, L., Pegg, R. B., Eitenmiller, R. R., Chun, J., Kerrihard, A. L. (2017). Selected nutrient analyses of fresh, fresh-stored, and frozen fruits and vegetables. *Journal of Food Composition and Analysis*, 59, 8–17. doi: 10.1016/j.jfca.2017.02.002.

[14] Bouzari, A., Holstege, D., Barrett, D. M. (2015). Vitamin Retention in Eight Fruits and Vegetables: A Comparison of Refrigerated and Frozen Storage. *Journal of Agricultural and Food Chemistry*, 63(3), 957–962. doi: 10.1021/jf5058793.

[15] Miller, S. R., Knudson, W. A. (2014). Nutrition and Cost Comparisons of Select Canned, Frozen, and Fresh Fruits and Vegetables. *American Journal of Lifestyle Medicine*, 8(6), 430–437. doi: 10.1177/1559827614522942.

[16] Dewanto, V., Wu, X., Adom, K. K., Liu, R. H. (2002). Thermal processing enhances the nutritional value of tomatoes by increasing total antioxidant activity. *Journal of Agricultural and Food Chemistry*, 50(10), 3010–3014. doi: 10.1021/jf0115589.

[17] European Chemicals Agency (2017, June 16). MSC unanimously agrees that Bisphenol A is an endocrine disruptor. Retrieved July 20, 2018 from https://echa.europa.eu/-/msc-unanimously-agrees-that-bisphenol-a-is-an-endocrine-disruptor.

[18] Haytowitz, D. B. (2011). Effect of draining and rinsing on the sodium and water soluble vitamin content of canned vegetables. *The FASEB Journal*, 25(1), 609.3.

[19] Lakkakula, A., Geaghan, J., Zanovec, M., Pierce, S., Tuuri, G. (2010). Repeated taste exposure increases liking for vegetables

by low-income elementary school children. *Appetite*, 55(2), 226–231. doi: 10.1016/j.appet.2010.06.003.

[20] Fritts, J. R., et al. (2018). Herbs and spices increase liking and preference for vegetables among rural high school students. *Food Quality and Preference*, 68, 125–134. doi: 10.1016/j.foodqual.2018.02.013.

[21] Peters, J. C., Polsky, S., Stark, R., Zhaoxing, P., Hill, J. O. (2014). The influence of herbs and spices on overall liking of reduced fat food. *Appetite*, 79, 183–188. doi: 10.1016/j.appet.2014.04.019.

[22] Tapsell, L. C., et al. (2006). Health benefits of herbs and spices: the past, the present, the future. *The Medical Journal of Australia*. 185, S4–24.

[23] Lim, S. S., et al. (2012). A comparative risk assessment of burden of disease and injury attributable to 67 risk factors and risk factor clusters in 21 regions, 1990–2010: a systematic analysis for the Global Burden of Disease Study 2010. *Lancet*, 380(9859), 2224–2260. doi: 10.1016/S0140-6736(12)61766-8.

[24] World Health Organization (2016, June 30). Salt reduction. Retrieved August 11, 2018 from http://www.who.int/news-room/fact-sheets/detail/salt-reduction.

[25] Granato, D., Branco, G. F., Nazzaro, F., Cruz, A. G., Faria, J. A. F. (2010). Functional Foods and Nondairy Probiotic Food Development: Trends, Concepts, and Products. *Comprehensive Reviews in Food Science and Food Safety*, 9(3), 292—302. doi: 10.1111/j.1541-4337.2010.00110.x.

[26] Smith-Spangler, C., et al. (2012). Are Organic Foods Safer or Healthier Than Conventional Alternatives?: A Systematic Review. *Annals of Internal Medicine*, 157(5), 348–366. doi: 10.7326/0003-4819-157-5-201209040-00007.

[27] Longo, V. D., Mattson, M. P. (2014). Fasting: Molecular Mechanisms and Clinical Applications. *Cell Metabolism,* 19(2), 181–192. doi: 10.1016/j.cmet.2013.12.008.

Made in the USA
Lexington, KY
03 May 2019